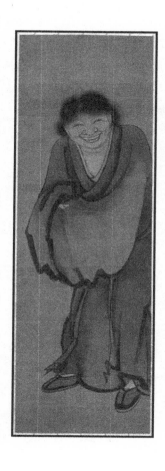

Gray House By Cold Mountain

GEORGE THOMAS

Yan Hui, *Han Shan* 寒山. Color on silk.
Tokyo National Museum

authorHOUSE®

AuthorHouse™
1663 Liberty Drive
Bloomington, IN 47403
www.authorhouse.com
Phone: 1-800-839-8640

Every character in this book is an authentic persona who
inhabits the realm of my fantasy life.

First published by AuthorHouse 8/9/2010

ISBN: 978-1-4520-2123-2 (e)
ISBN: 978-1-4520-2122-5 (sc)

Library of Congress Control Number: 2010908809

Printed in the United States of America
Bloomington, Indiana

This book is printed on acid-free paper.

For all characters, fictional and real, living or dead,
whose unforgettable reality have formed shapes in the synaptic
landscape inside my skull—I thank you.

Special appreciation and love for both *Big* (who recently succumbed
to cancer) and *Little* (a creative inspiration) *Geoff*, the 12 Step crew in
Spokane who sailed with me over a long distance before I jumped ship
(as opposed to falling off the wagon) and, until death us do part, many
rapturous hugs for my wife, Mertie, whose nurturance soothes me and who
does not find any of the material in this book to be pornographic.

Acknowledgment and thanks to Gary Snyder for his emotive translations of Han-shan's work which inspired me as I holed up in the little gray house on Cannon Street in 1993 and to Robert B. Henricks whose translations of the same poet's work gave me the prosaic style that my own 8-line poems took on as I wrote them.

The poetry is selected from two unpublished manuscripts of poetry. Three—62, 71 and 81(from *Secrets Of Cold Mountain*) appeared in *EIDOS*.

Contents

Selections from COLD MOUNTAIN VISIONS OF OLD GRAYHOUSE — 1
Cold Mountain Visions of Old Grayhouse

Selections from SECRETS OF COLD MOUNTAIN — 35
Secrets Of Cold Mountain

Selections from
COLD MOUNTAIN VISIONS OF OLD GRAYHOUSE

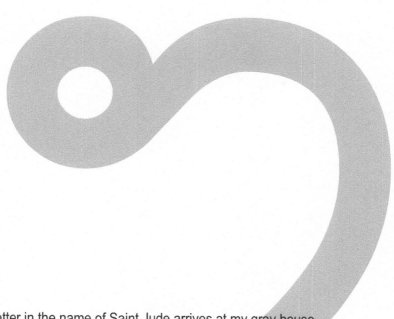

[1]

A letter in the name of Saint Jude arrives at my gray house,
Promising good fortune—a better job, health, beautiful wife—
But I must forward twenty copies within four days. If I fail,
My fortune will turn bad. I'll lose my job, be loveless, go blind!
One poor fellow in Uruguay was eaten by army ants!
Another in Chile was chopped into a chili! A reasonable man,
I consider my ten dollar couch, my gall bladder scar,
My empty bed and wonder how I missed that earlier letter!

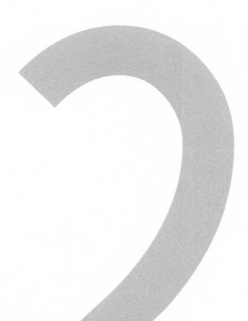

[2]

Sometimes I travel out from my gray cave
On Cannon Street into the larger world. Human voices
Fill my ringing ears, car sounds, malls where
Hundreds of steel steeds sit between yellow lines.
Momentarily confused, I think my realm is there,
Lighted fluorescent—red, orange, green and blue.
Strange heaven where an appetite never rests, hungry
For meat at the Red Robin hamburger emporium.

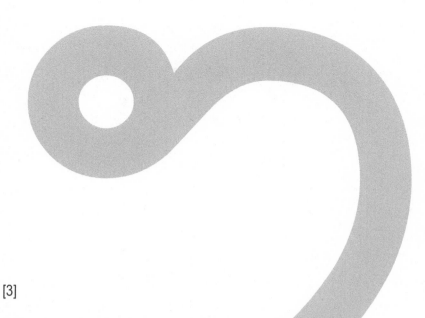

[3]

This is not Cold Mountain I see, not Han-shan.
I'm not a wild man poet nor one of the Immortals.
I dwell in a little gray place on Cannon Street,
Just right for one man wise enough to be alone.
After years of wandering and three wives,
Like Zorba I can say, "...the whole catastrophe!"
But I must admit to it three times. In the flight path
Overhead, combat jets whoop it up like cranes.

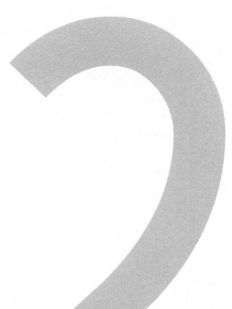

[4]

Unlike Han-shan, no remote cliff face to carve my graffiti on,
Old Gray-house makes do with the backs of used computer paper
Stolen home from work. On one side, numerical control programs
Which keep the wheels of industry grinding; on the other,
Whatever my muse happens to stumble across. I'm in a race
With the wheels of industry to see which will wear out first.
Late in the century for me, I eat lots of inexpensive pasta,
Pondering when the damn computers will run out of numbers.

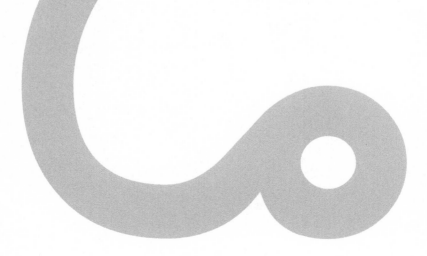

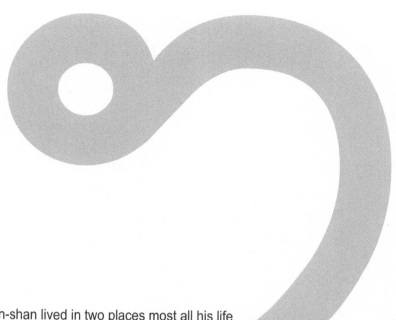

[6]

Han-shan lived in two places most all his life
Whereas, at one time, Old Grayhouse worked fifty-three
Jobs in a space of thirty years. Florida swamps,
Ohio forests, Washington scabland—road dust in a rear vision mirror,
New vistas over and old again, the only constant
Being.... Now I've come to settle in this small
Gray cave on Cannon Street, but, as after daylong drives,
The road still an itch in the seat of my pants.

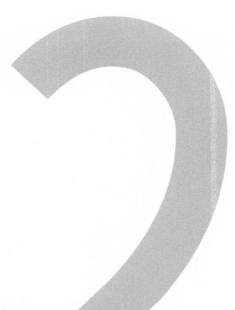

[7]

As for me, I delight in the everyday Way—waking,
Brushing my teeth, going off to work, the lovely snarl
Of traffic and gentle drivers, the refreshing mountains
Of polluted air, the roads to work varied and twisted,
Accessible and easily traveled on rubber sandals from Akron.
If I'm lucky I get through the day with my senses intact,
The angry Genie of America will leave one of these utterances
For me to find on my pillow some mornings when I wake.

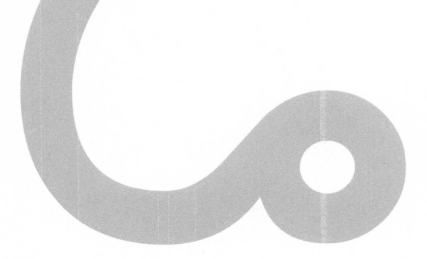

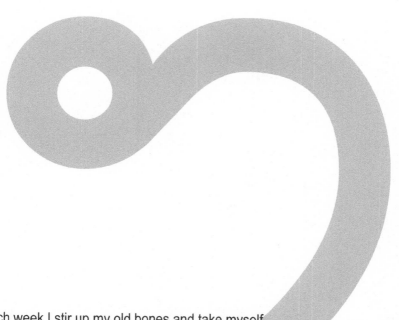

[8]

Each week I stir up my old bones and take myself
To meetings. There, as fragments of the same spirit,
We share the small ways we keep our demons bottled up.
Fortuitously, we discover vistas of happiness within.
If one is not careful, however, he may come
To think too much of happiness. In that bottle,
A real American genie hides beside the road. One can
Get carried away by all the snake oil salesmen selling it.

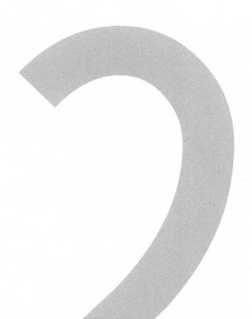

[9]

Bad gas tints orange the sky along the ridges of this valley city.
Through geometries of brick and glass, iron steeds farting clouds
Of death, old Gray-house strolls uneasily to McDonald's breakfast.
He craves people, wants to listen to canned, easy-rocking music.
There, where lost saxophones wail out of their jazz element, he observes
A city from which all poets have been accidentally excluded.
Han-shan, so many centuries earlier, could you have imagined
This emptiness? Man-mountain, where is my place in all of this?

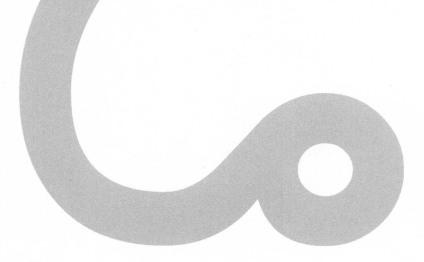

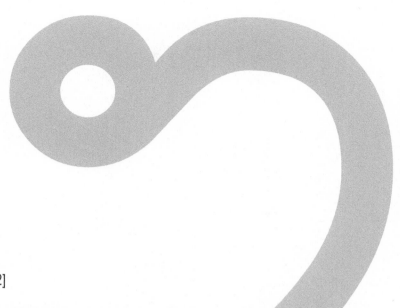

[12]

Woman! Now there's a universe for you!
A pretentious male in a silly French movie said,
"The bodies of women are incredible!" I know
The hazards of that Way—a man can never grow old
In peace. Alone with my varicose leg, my
Bifocal vision, I clump through this lifetime of mine,
Still wearing the essence of my calamity—the
Indelible mystery of women—like a Venusian perfume.

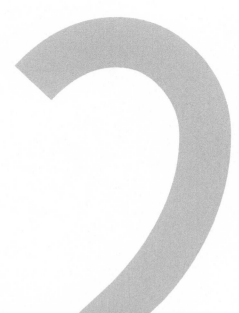

[13]

Let the worldly ones shoulder each other aside
In the bull markets of the great metropolises.
These great ones can laugh at me since I mock myself too.
They have my permission. I admit I cut a very minor
Figure as the world goes, a poor poet, inveterate scribbler,
A dreamer, mostly deaf to the shouts of the marketplace,
But it's hard to be humble when I know myself
To be the most perfect fool who ever lived.

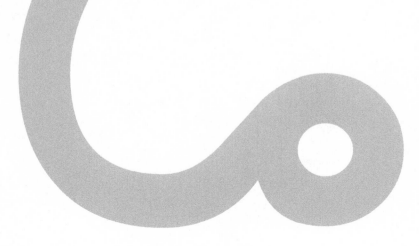

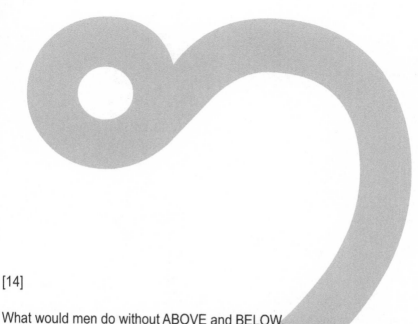

[14]

What would men do without ABOVE and BELOW,
Without UP or DOWN? What would men do for direction?
Mountains are TALL and imposing, valleys DEEP
And treacherous. We look DOWN on knaves and fools,
And women grow UP to be wise and nurturing mothers.
Can it be true as the dead Prophet suggested
That there is wisdom in becoming "as little children"?
A medium-short gnome, I ponder these mysteries.

[15]

This bed of mine gives me pleasure—nothing more than
A sleeping bag folded once, a sheet thrown over,
Topped off with a delightfully pink electric blanket.
I used to awake in a real bed, but it was borrowed, and
The lender took it back. She needs all three of her bedrooms
Furnished, she says, though no one visits her. She drinks and
In her cups has a shrewish temperament. Her selfishness is perfect—
Awakening mornings, I sit up, my low bed an instant prayer rug

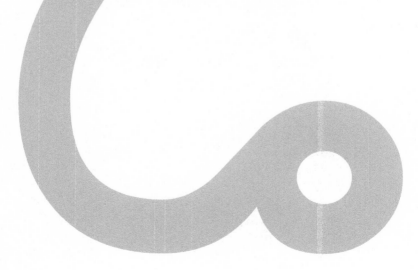

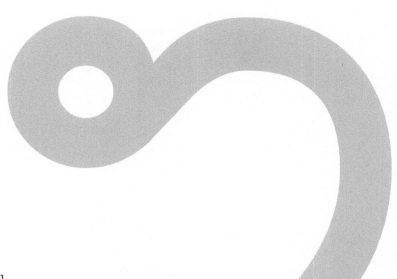

[16]

This old-fashioned tub with lion paw feet!
I sit in it, Han-shan, a stranger to myself,
Un-centered, miserly in a small, gray house,
A failure by all accounting methods—a toyless
Potentate, sarcastic, washing my own back,
Painfully contorting my frail body to reach it.
Perhaps I should invest in a back scrubber,
But that would cost me my exquisite pain!

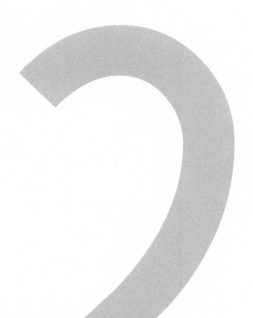

[17]

A lion-pawed tub is quite a vessel to travel in! Voyeur,
I stand outside my bathroom doorway to watch myself bathe—
Face, ears, arms, chest, penis, ass, legs, toes, hair.
Who is that old man, what is he thinking of in his body parts?
Certainly not centered, Han-shan, like you under your white top.
Outside himself, beyond himself, asleep in himself, how many
Thousand times has he anointed that body with washing ritual?
His thoughts whirling like autumn leaves, where is his rubber ducky?

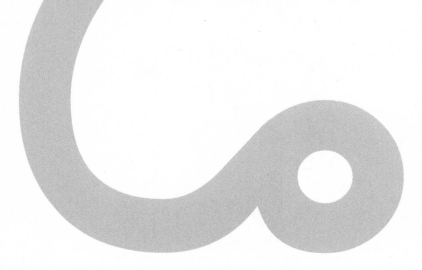

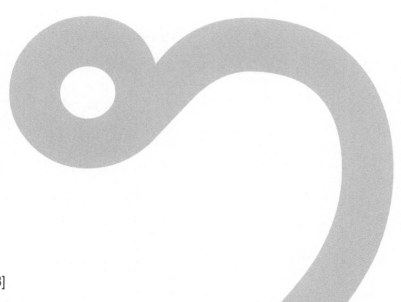

[18]

People ask the way to my old gray house
On Cannon Street. A foolish question!
So many streets lead here, as many ways as people
Who travel them. You can get this way from anywhere.
Seasons come and go, days and nights pass, all
Leading to the same conclusion: click your red shoe
Heels together three times, stay close within your skin,
And soon you'll imagine that you're here!

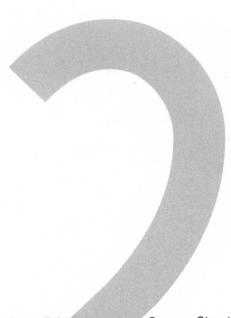

[19]

Wonderful to be here in my little gray cave on Cannon Street,
Smelling of five days without a bath. From here I can imagine
The Castle-On-A-Hill, its brilliantly lighted windows, beckoning
Across the snow. Inside—lit tapers, gleaming silver,
Crisp napkins folded as swans, plates in neat order, music
Of the day, polite conversation—all as regular and calm as
A funeral procession. Nose pressed against the window of my
Gray place, armpits reeking, a secret joy transforms my heart.

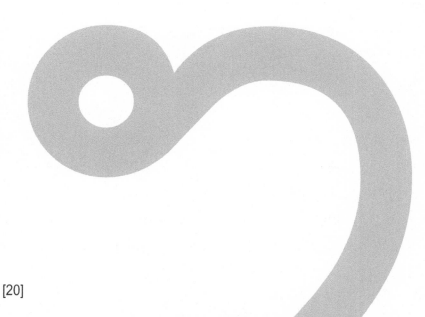

[20]

Bukowski and Kerouac, Snyder, Camus and Han-shan, lounging
Beside a mountain pool—I wave to them. Then here comes Woody
Along the path with his woeful shtick of failed relationships,
His puzzled frown which says, "We don't know. We never will!"
He's so far away from Cold Mountain, Han-shan, from my fantasy
Of the clear mountain pool which, centered in my dream,
Reflects your sage white head. See how he, his naked dialogue
From a sexual scene, stumbles in to disturb its placid surface?

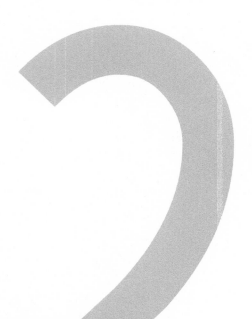

[22]

Workshop poems are the truth in jail! I could go on
With this image of jail and write a workshop poem, but
I'm interrupted by a dog barking several houses down
In the dark backyard where he's prowling. I
Listen to my neighbor's lawn sprinkler, I enjoy the cool,
Midnight air on my hairy, fat, bare belly. Been
A long, hot June day that's burned my bald head red.
With jails everywhere, I rub my fat Buddha belly and glow.

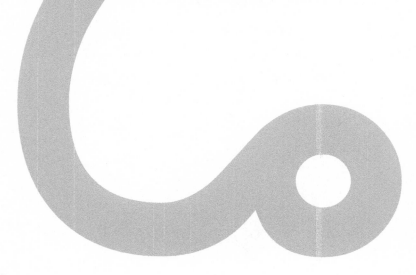

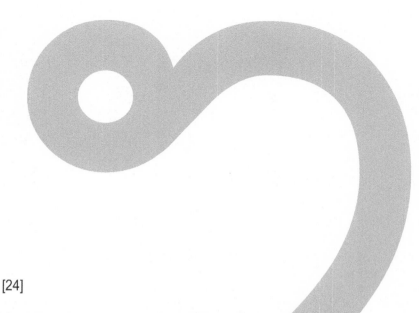

[24]

Sage Han-shan grew reclusive in his old age.
Retiring into the airiness of his mountain retreats,
He left behind the empty husks of the ancient texts,
Confined to fragile memory the perfume of young women.
He walked solitary beside the towering peak of Cold Mountain
And knew himself to be safely within the Beautiful Eye of Heaven.
Old Gray-house should be so wise who prowls the supermarket
Aisles in search of heavenly eye contact with passing beauty.

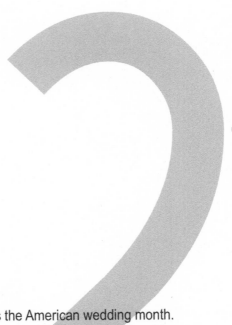

[26]

Traditionally, June is the American wedding month.
The bride comes down the aisle in something old,
Something new, something borrowed, something blue.
The groom's not to see the bride before the wedding hour.
As for me, it's three times up and three times struck out
At the old altar game. When it comes to marriage, a sage
Might well think to toss a coin: "heads" it works, "tails" I lose.
Some sorry-ass wise men should never see the bride.

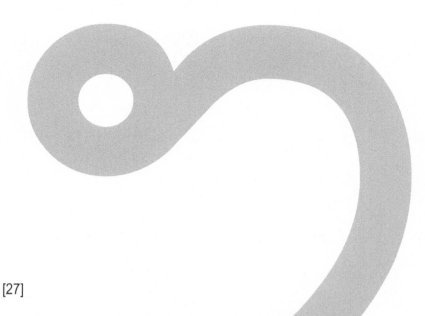

[27]

Who is that old man twelve rows back from the screen,
Sitting alone with a book of Han-shan's poetry in his lap?
Around him, loving couples hold hands, families share popcorn.
Old Baldy is barren at the very peak, but his long side hair is drawn
Back in a pony tail. Dim theater lights reflect off his shiny dome.
While he waits, he tries to read Han-shan in the gloom.
The movie begins—"Last of the Mohicans" with Daniel Day-Lewis.
His mind leaps centuries in a single bound. He cries with joy!

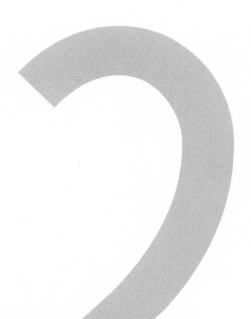

[28]

What is this fog that licks against my gray walls and hides
The sun, shrivels my wildflowers in a killing frost?
Cold drizzle falls on October streets, walking makes me shiver.
Some New Age thinkers believe weather can affect our moods,
Some say we are the pawns of planetary alignments. Ha!
If only my fate were that easy to unravel, gladly
I'd reach up and shift the orbits of the Earth and stars,
But this drizzly mist just swallows up my flailing fists.

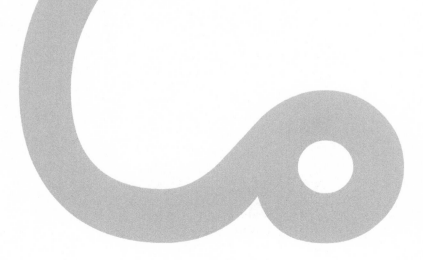

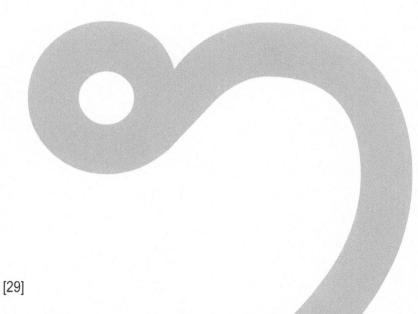

[29]

Gray man in a gray house in a gray world, ask yourself,
Why continue in this old way, silly Scribbler? Out there,
In the great world, no one hears of you. What you do is of
No earthly use to the average man bent upon his worldly task.
Gray man, your ghost haunts imaginary banquets of fame—
Inconspicuously by the wall, hands shielding its genitals,
It hears mocking laughter as, bent over empty paper like
One of Pavlov's dogs, you fill space with endless slaver.

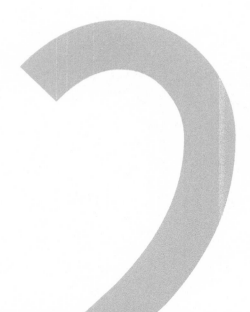

[30]

Mid-fifties, an awkward age. The young women who bring my meals
Stroke my arm affectionately. They don't seem to see the *real* me.
Confused, I don't know whether these beauties who touch my shoulder
Are placating an old bull or see me as a gentle father, a good tipper
Or a potentially gentle lover. Always juvenile, what do I know of sex!
If I cross the line and declare myself, will they scream, "Dirty old man!"
Or grant me a boon? Han-shan, long before the daze of Freud, should
I ask now or retreat forever to my gray shack by Cold Mountain?

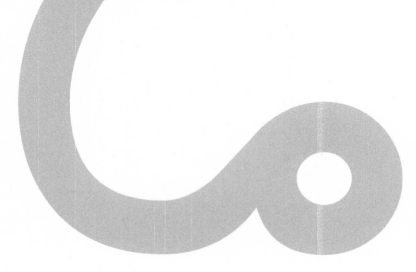

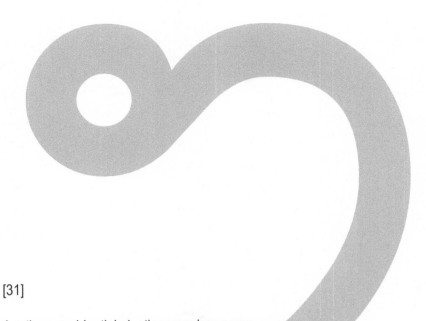

[31]

Another presidential election year has come
And gone. The boisterous claims fall silent.
These men we elect to manage our public affairs
Have reached (with many promises) the banquets of power.
Each claims to want the very best for us, each
Promises to have all the answers to our questions.
Here, in my little gray house on Cannon Street,
I struggle to decide "fish" or "fowl" for lunch.

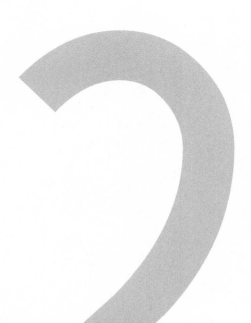

[32]

Winter gray mornings in my gray house on Cannon Street,
If I read or if I pray, spirits come to haunt me.
Meister Ekhardt came this morning into my bedroom.
"The seed of God is growing inside you into God," he said.
I don't know what to make of it! Will this growth shove
My organs aside to make room, lift my heart a few inches
And sink my intestines? I'm so full of gut and gore,
I can only imagine a lifelong carcinoma growing in there.

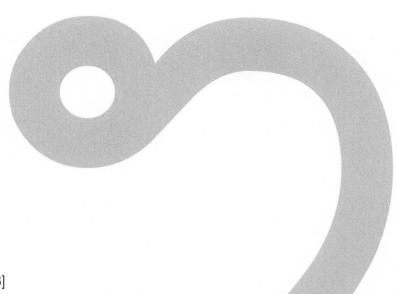

[33]

When old Han-shan of the Tang Dynasty, walking dusty roads,
Describes shy girls with silken sleeves and chignons
Pinned with ducks of jade, the predictable critics
Comment on the "wistful nature" of the old poet's later work.
What will they say of the late Twentieth Century work
Of Old Grayhouse who sits in the music-loud, Deja Vu dark
To watch young girls strip naked on a stage and pays
Twelve dollars to have one sit and wiggle on his lap?

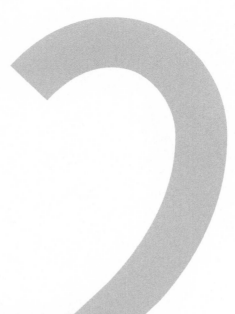

[35]

Last night she was dark rather than light,
And my questions disturbed her in the gloom.
Deja Vu dancer who didn't wish to share her history
With a stranger, she was troubled by lustful youths.
"They see only my beauty. It's nothing! There's more
To me than what they see. My life in this place is only a tiny
Fraction of who I am." Old man, shriveling like a prune,
I stare into beauty's eyes, bemused by beauty's troubles.

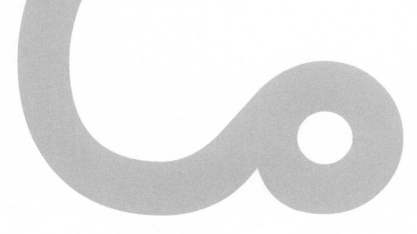

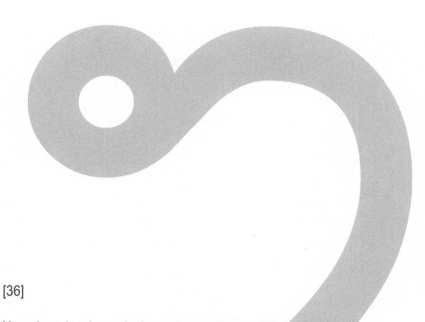

[36]

Han-shan, I wake early these days, my eyes full of grit,
My ears of silence. Puffing with exertion, I push myself upright
And seize my pen, intending to send a piece of anger into the world.
Then I realize the darkness I'm sitting in. It's so dark I must turn
On a light to see to write. For a moment I think of all poets
Out there in this dark with me and those on the other side,
Turning together on a solitary globe in dark space,
Me, Old Grayhouse, my front door just now entering the light.

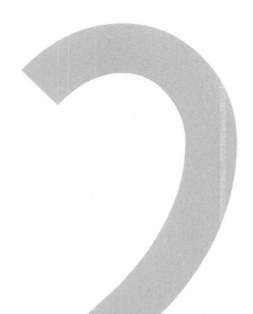

[38]

New Year 1992. Mr. Double Nickel has witnessed many changes,
Passing along the beat path through foothills to visit Cold Mountain.
Of old intellectual friends—F. Scott, Eugene, Papa, Henry, Fyodor,
Albert, Jack, Tennessee, doomed, addicted—not many survive.
Still in the flesh, others—Snyder, Ginsberg, Burroughs—do.
Watching gaunt Burroughs appear in junkie movies like a ghost,
Old Gray-house sits riveted in dark theaters, waiting for the figure
Of his own veiled ghost to appear, whistling up over the next hill.

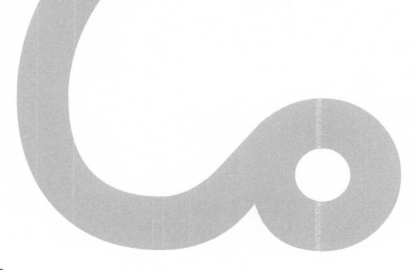

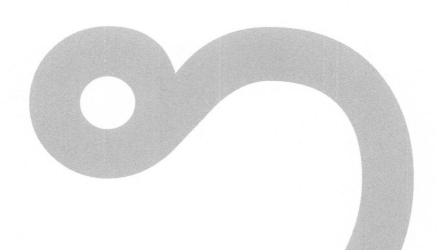

[40]

Young. All of them have the hourglass figures of nymphs,
And these girls of the Deja Vu will dance naked for you
Up on a stage. For so many dollars more, they'll give you
A *Texas couch dance*, climb up to sit on your lap and wiggle
Until you come. All this in a dark, windowless room
Far from the small, safe gray house you call home.
Foolish, gray-haired codger with boyish desires, why fret?
Even as dark angels sit on your lap, there is growth.

Selections from
SECRETS OF COLD MOUNTAIN

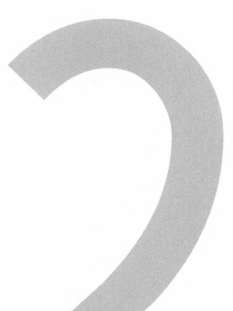

[42]

I want to fuck you in darkness and light.
I want to push myself deep into your steaming asshole.
I want to listen to your shuddering moans of pleasure under me,
The gasped in-drawing of your breath, the whimper
Of your pursed lips. I want to feel the returning thrust
Of your soft ass cheeks into my hard hip bones.
While my heart pounds with this exercise of strife and love,
Losing all my painful memories in you must be a heaven like this.

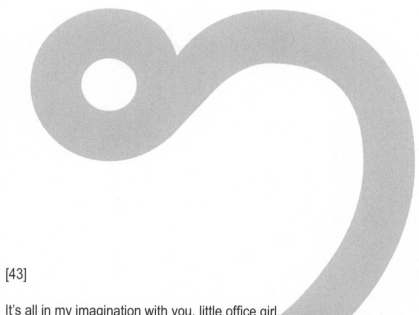

[43]

It's all in my imagination with you, little office girl.
Maybe always will be. I enjoy the curves of your ass
Stretching the tight Levis you wear. I watch your big jugs
Shift beneath your sweaters, can imagine how they'd swing
Beneath you if we do it from behind, how they'd sway before my eyes
If you sit above me. I can imagine you, tensed, sitting on me,
Closed eyes, seeking your release, while I, below, hang on every moan,
Every whimper, hang like a school boy on every swing of your big jugs.

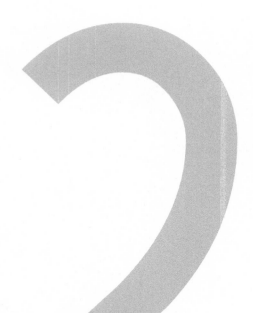

[45]

What a delight it is to stand naked with you before this full length mirror,
To have you bend at the waist and take me into your willing mouth,
To feel your warm breath bathing the length of my wet shaft.
What a view of heaven I have in your spreading buttocks,
Shaped like a cloven hoof or the globe after a cosmic event!
So animal is my delight, your ass could be the ass of a cow, a sheep,
The ass of any animal I might be lustful enough to approach, but they
Don't have warm fingers to creep between my legs and tickle my balls!

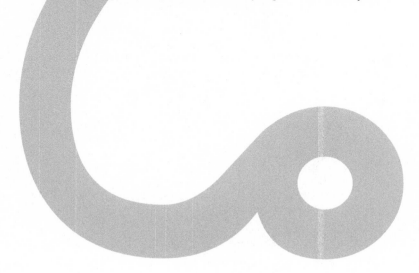

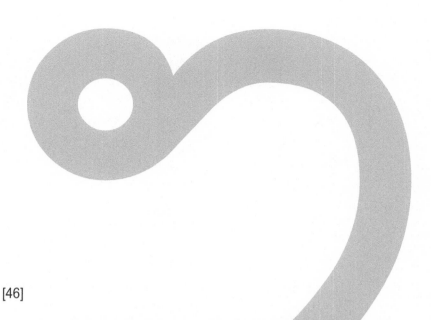

[46]

You were the first, secretive and demur like any woman of the Fifties.
Unless your were a bit tipsy, you'd pretend not to be eager, not
A part of what we did! O how I loved it in the living room with you,
Where I'd lead you to lay your trim bare butt on the Early American cloth.
Your head on the couch arm, your eyes closed, you awaited my pleasure,
Then I'd put one of your feet down on the floor and raise your other leg
To the couch back until you were spread before me like an unread book!
Obsessed, I lay between your legs to plunge my tongue into your shy secrets.

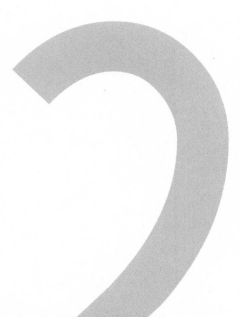

[49]

She's the one I still most dream of, with her needs that drove her to please.
While her pensive eyes watched, to fetch from the closet shelf our hidden
Collection of soft cloth belts, to spread and tie her like a cipher on the sheet,
To shove a pillow under her contracting buttocks, then to nip and nuzzle
over every ridge and valley of her fragrant body. This was earthly paradise!
I would lick her up and down, straddle her and push my snake between
Her nuzzling lips until her urgent cries and circling hips told me it was time
To scramble up where the spring gushed and plunge in, wildly bleating.

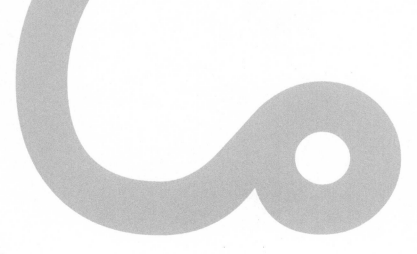

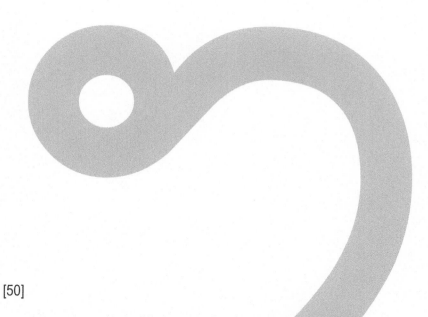

[50]

Such delicious ambiguity to be a child in your house, to receive
The enemas you regularly shoved into my tight boyish bunghole.
They yielded the same ambiguous pain as your beatings. Those
Enigmatic times confused me, like the time in puberty I lay at foot
Of your marriage bed to watch a new-fangled TV, its small screen
Opening the whole world to me. Glancing back, I saw your flexed knees
Wide under the cotton nightgown. Your naked truth made me breathless.
Our eyes met, you silent. All my life since I lay at the foot of your bed.

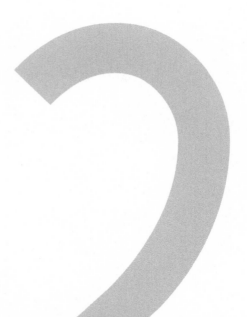

[52]

That 1950s one—she was hard to get off, and I was young and quick.
The bare thought of her virgin sheath around my love tool finished me!
O! I worked so hard to do my duty, good little boy that I was,
Waiting, waiting my turn, holding back. Fore-playing like a fiend,
I'd finger and probe her tight slit, then get down in there with my tongue.
Later, my chin dripping, I'd slurp love juices over her swollen nipples.
Sometimes, I'd lie on my back and slide under/between her kneeling legs,
Like under a car, to work on her starter button with my busy tongue wrench.

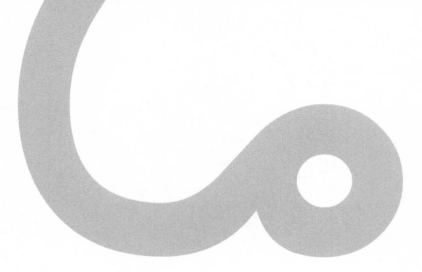

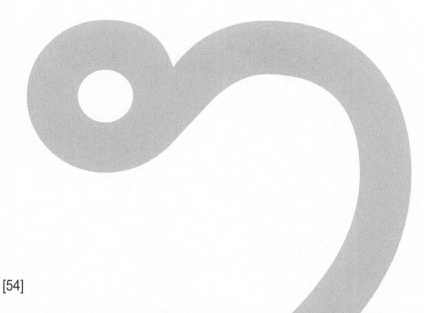

[54]

There were times we did this. I'd tie her dainty wrists behind her back
With a soft, bathrobe belt then lash her to the doorknob of the closet.
Standing there, cold, vulnerable, she'd close her eyes and thrust out
Her small breasts to be kissed and bitten. I'd rub my cock excitedly
Against her goose-bumped thigh, kiss and bite her neck, thrust my tongue
Into her mouth and suck on her fat lower lip. Moving lower, I'd take one
Of her titties in my stretched, hungry mouth and bite it till she whimpered.
After many times like that, eating my captive alive, I became her love slave.

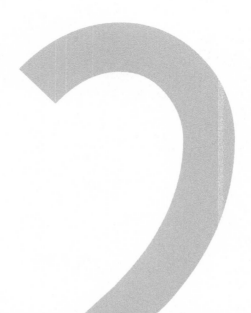

[55]

Why are they always separate? I never forget you, redheaded girl,
Our rendezvous in a mutual friend's apartment while that sad wife
In the outer world fretted with children and keeping up a house.
Pale thick legs and thin red curls between your virgin, Irish thighs,
I knew so little how to please but brought you Dowson's poems
And long night drives full of talk, pouring out my soul to you.
My spindly cock poking in your willing cunt was a failure. Your first
Orgasm gentle as a wish, I thought, *Is that all?* Was my soul enough?

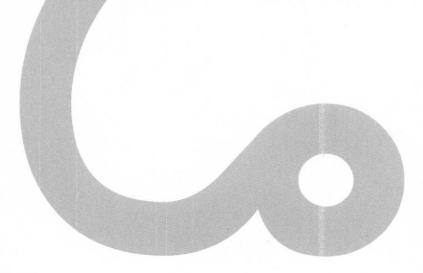

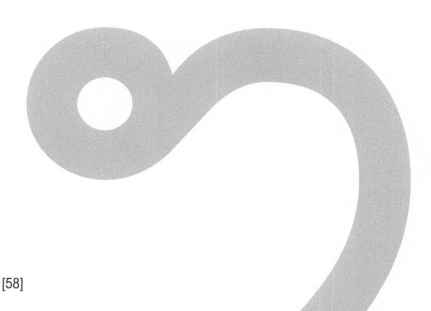

[58]

Though she was always bashful, she liked it that way too
Once I got her accustomed to it. First we'd go out for dinner
And dancing. A few drinks loosened her up. Pressing close,
I'd rub her trim, dancing butt under her tight skirt. Home
I'd strip her naked and roll her on her stomach and spread her legs.
Lovely ass upthrust, she'd lie there, eyes closed, a compliant but alert
    servant.
When I greased her up and entered by the rear door, she knew the master
Was home, wriggling and greeting him with enthusiastic cries of joy.

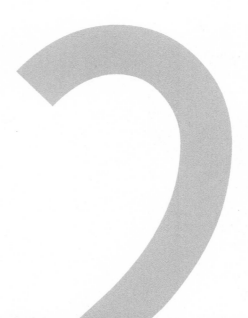

[59]

I'm captive now, remembering how you closed your eyes and sank
Into yourself to suck my cock between your red lips, trying
With all your wanton mouth to succor me, then, guided by my hands,
Turned on your knees, bending to accept me from the rear like a dog,
Your dark asshole exposed to take my finger to the second knuckle,
Small breasts dangling, a nipple brushing on my upturned palm,
Your clitoris responsive to my fingertip—all this in silence, intent,
A civil war, your whole body betraying your strongholds one by one.

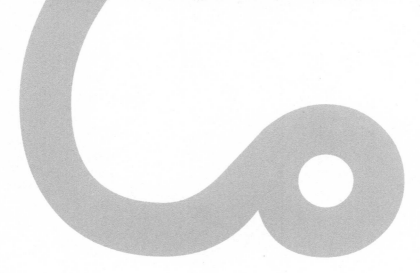

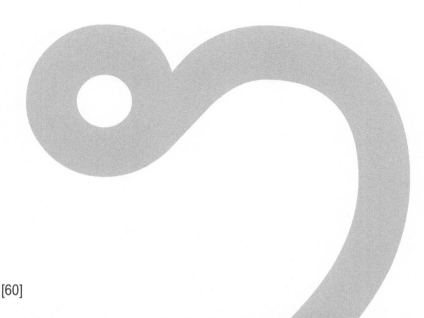

[60]

A young man can't appreciate a shy woman like a Grayhouse can—
What it is to lead a quiet one earnestly climbing to reach the peaks.
I remember one who used to pretend to sleep for the longest time
While my hand stole under the pliant waistband of her baby doll bottoms,
My fingers spread over cool, smooth skin to grasp her prim buttocks, the
Steamy warmth begin to rise out of the tight crack, the moist slit, slipping
My middle finger at last into the watering hole, all the while this shy
Tigress waiting for me to enter the bush so she could roar and pounce.

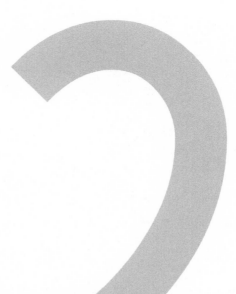

[61]

I harden, remembering the shy reserve of your love making, recalling now
The first time in the darkened bedroom after a few drinks and dancing
When I turned you to your smooth stomach and licked the butt hole sheltering
Within the hills of your ass. You waited pensively, as usual, with closed eyes,
Arms encircling the pink pillow beneath your head, while I slid up to stretch
My body over yours. Still teasing, you waited as I kissed your neck.
I heard your breath release when I pressed into the tight hole I'd prepared
With the spittle of my tongue. My fingers sought under your thighs for
The magic button. That's when you came suddenly alive, thrusting between
Delights like a church maiden just discovering the pleasures of hell.

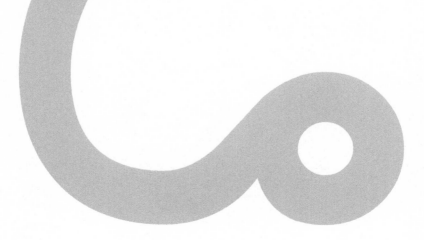

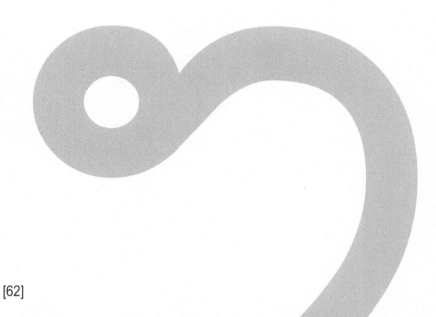

[62]

How I lust for the past, for the cloth belts around my wrists and ankles, to find
My legs tied helplessly wide on the bed sheets! Then I loved to study your
Intense, preoccupied look, watch your full ass cheeks spread, tits bobbling,
As you scurried to bend and tie me hand and foot. My normally hidden
Self swells up stiff, pointing to my dizzy head as if to say, "It's all lies!"
You straddle me, your hungry mouth opens, cheeks puff to gobble me down,
And I want a hand free to slip my finger up your ass and make you gasp with
Pleasure and wriggle giggle, but I'm helpless, tied in memory hand and foot.

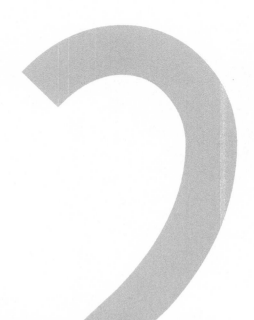

[63]

You laughed delightedly when I encapsulated my existence as *a lifetime*
Spent slaving over a hot body, but I can see you, my little Hotpoint,
On my countertop, your sudsy hands tied behind you, your tiny breasts
Thrusting up from your bony ribcage topped with nipples grown the size
And texture of wine corks under the pulling of my thirsty lips. My nimble
Fingers fiddle with your knobs, turn up the heat. Your eyes glow with
The emptiness that burns within you. When I climb up to insert a modest
Meat loaf, my heart sinks, wondering where I'll find the next course.

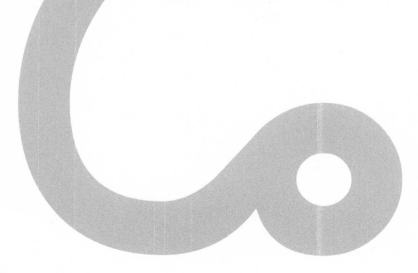

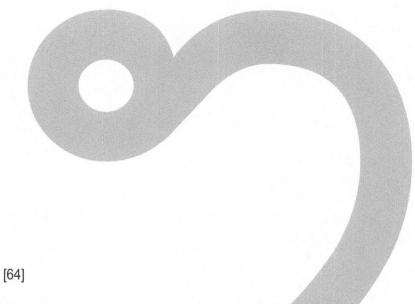

[64]

At an age I can't play half court anymore, my libido has gone
Inactive. Since August I've been dormant, dead as an old volcano.
Yet there you are, a flirtatious waitress with a tight behind,
Round as a basketball, walking on pipe stem legs, frizzy auburn hair
In bouncy, tightly coiled rings. You're gangly as a colt as I watch
Your bottom wiggling over wiping one of your tables at work.
I slip you out of your shorts and, spreading you, erupt with thoughts
Of balancing your basketball on the tip of my index finger.

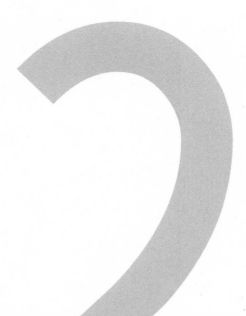

[66]

I still grow short of breath when I think of your puzzling shyness, still
Make rare drives by your house, hoping to glimpse your dainty fingers.
I remember our last time, me on my side, my cheek pillowed on
Your satin thigh, my busy tongue. Down at the other end were you,
Lips as busy with me as mine with you, our heads eagerly bobbing
To gobble. Then your surprising assault, burning in my rear!
Later, amused with yourself, you lifted that finger and tasted it.
Even now, this asshole craves your anal humor.

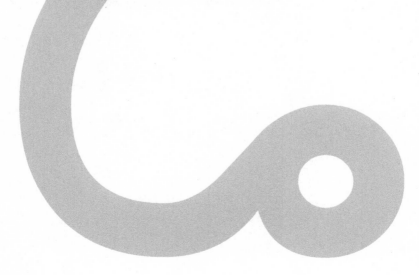

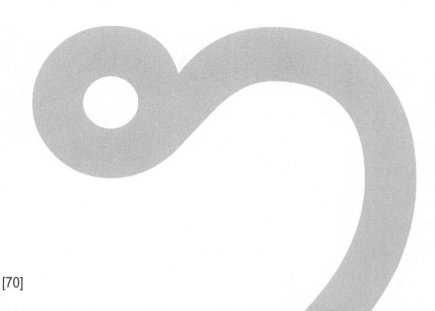

[70]

Let me count one way: together we stand, facing a full length mirror,
Me behind and rubbing my cock between your fleshy cheeks. My hands
Play along your ribcage, up over your small breasts, their hardening nipples.
My fingers trace down your belly which arches like a cat's back; they slip
    between
Your thighs to stroke the tumescent labia. Your knees flex. Moaning, you reach
Behind to grip my cock in your small, cool fingers. My turn to moan.
I run my full eyes over your trapped figure in the mirror. "Look at us!"
I urge, but you only peek between slit lids and seize my balls.

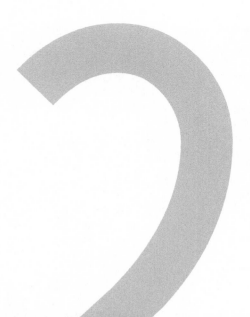

[71]

You are long ago gone, another man commands your willing ass.
My mind inevitably invades the bedroom which is yours and his
To hear your abandoned groans, your ravenous thrusting under him.
Why must I remember women so strongly and always kneeling
Before me or, 69, above or beneath me with my cock
Thrust deeply in their mouths? You were always sucking me off,
Your mouth ever willing to please me and my stiff projections.
When will I have my fill of it, the way you eat me alive?

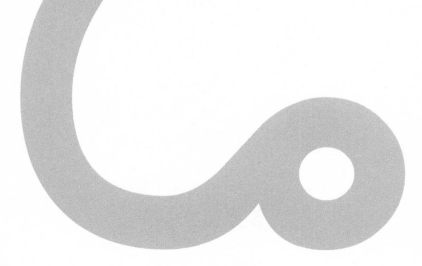

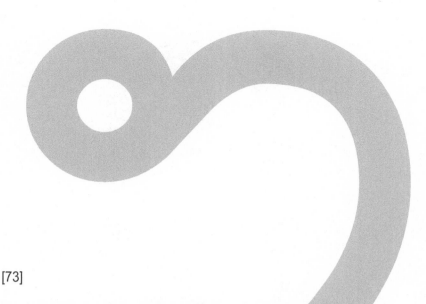

[73]

Memories come with me in the morning out of dreams. I awake,
Remembering how I straddled you and pressed my ass to your lips,
And face to ass between your legs, pulled your legs back
Under my arms, rolling your bottom right up into my mouth
Where I licked you hole to hole, then, commanding your two
Fingers under mine, pressed them into yourself until we were two
Masturbating one. Growing wild with you, my lips and chin coated
With you, I got another finger in and my tongue.
Later I ate your fingers like juicy steaks. All this gluttony!
But not enough to fill an old man mourning for his youth.

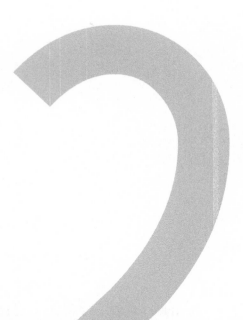

[74]

For months I contemplated a slim green cucumber and your comely twat,
Thought of its ribs, how they would tickle all its length into you,
Considered if it should be cool to make your nipples stand or be inserted
Room temperature for comfort, and burned, anticipating how I would slip
From the bed while you waited in the dark and, returning, make you raise and
Spread your knees as I press it in, watch you suspiciously watch it enter you.
When finally you wantonly stir to receive it, I savor your joyous cries, later,
While you contentedly smile, suck your juices off it as gay as you please.

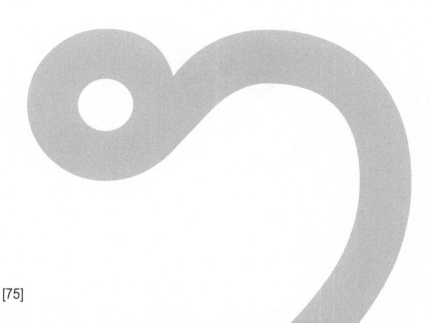

[75]

You were very exciting, the way your willing body said, *I love you so!*
You would put your mouth anywhere I liked, open any orifice to me.
I could place your cunt face down and cheeks ass up to receive me—
Tongue, cock or dildo, cucumber or banana, angry, sad, soft or grinding
Into the anywhere of you I liked. I commanded you, my obedient slave,
To *Open Sesame* and, in the blink of an eye, you opened, always willing!
Happy, sad, angry, lonely, pensive, reluctant or gay, you were always ready till,
Sated, I withdrew and you fled to another, leaving me to feel like such a dildo!

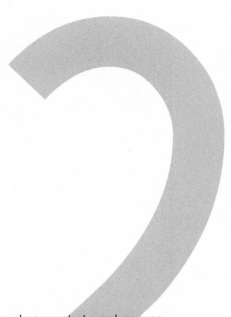

[78]

So it's your mouth now I concentrate on because
The day shift tells me you've got a "real mouth" on you.
I can imagine a tirade of your curses streaming out:
"O fuck, O fuck, O fuck me, fuck me, fuck..," and my sides
Aching as I breathlessly pump my bone into you doggy style,
My loins slamming into your hard-boned, stretched flanks,
Striving desperately, straining to empty you of curses,
Praying for nothing but sweetness on your tongue.

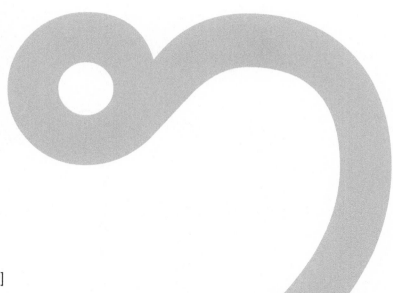

[79]

Now it seems to be your turn in my poems when fear strikes at work again.
I don't know what to make of this balloon of ache in the groin that rises
From way down low up into my throat like a blues wail when I think of you
In the next office. Is it fear of getting what I want—your body bent to mine?
The day shift says you've quite the mouth on you. They mean language, but
I think of you kneeling before me, your lips rounded to accept my difficult
Philosophy or, kneeling breast to breast, I run my fingers between your thighs,
And your sweet, red lips open to my lips to accept my tongue, my words.

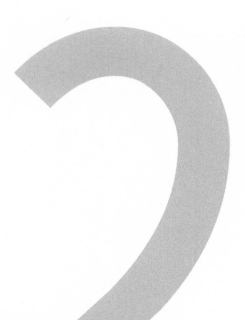

[81]

I was titillated when you, my giggling, brown Italian Beatrice,
Your undulant labia purplish as grape skins, your dark nipples round
And firm as mushroom stems, told me your fantasy, to wit—to lick
Whipped cream from my balls and shove a candle up my ass. Thus
Aroused, desirous of your favor, I lay postulant, legs spread, and felt
Your tongue's adoration of my balls while with a stubby, white
Devotional candle you worshiped at my puckered ass. Later, Dante
Returned from hell, I threw myself at your dainty feet to suck your big toes.

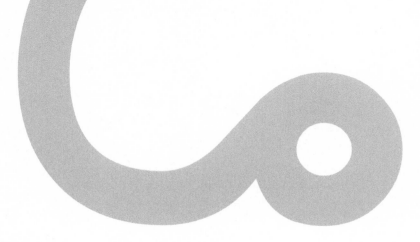

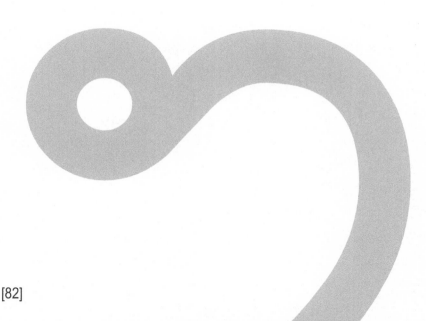

[82]

I love language, and you weren't bashful either when I led you naked
To the living room and sat your full bottom on the soft, grape-colored
Couch arm in the darkness and lay you back until, shoulders resting
On seat cushions, your ass in air, you were exposed. There I knelt
To your secrets, lip level before me, and lowered my face to feast with
Tongue and lips on the sweetness hidden there in those two springs,
And when I dipped a finger into this or that one, my exploratory probes
Set your heels to dancing, your lips to speaking tongues.

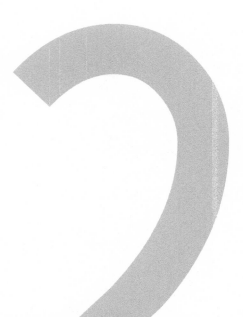

[83]

A dog's life to be so old and watch your sweet, young ass in Levis strut
Out the door and know I'll never fuck you. Those two round globes
Of flesh, sausages in blue casings, that bounce and jiggle hide two small
Holes I want to probe—one with my ding dong and one with my finger—
Until I hear you cry and holler and bite your lower lip while your face
Falls apart and thighs start to tremble. Watching you, I want to get
Down on hands and knees and poke my nose between your legs, follow you
Out the door, sniffing, while you wiggle and giggle and push at my snout.

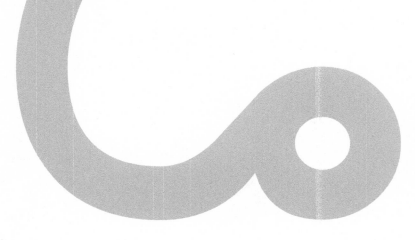

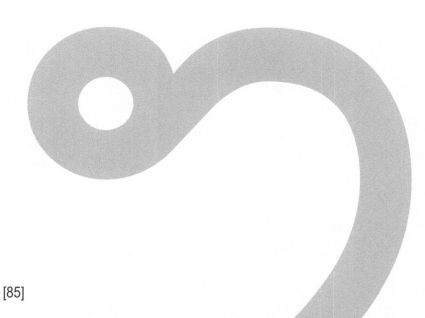

[85]

I want to lavish my tongue around and around one of your nipples
Until it swells to an olive. I want to engulf one of your
Small breasts in my mouth and suck its rubbery toughness
Until my jaws ache, arching my spine, pull my head back
And stretch your sweet flesh until you moan with pleasure
And pain. Plunging my hard life into your hot, yielding center,
O body of young love and sweet desire, let me fill my eyes,
My nose, my hungry mouth with memories of my mortality!

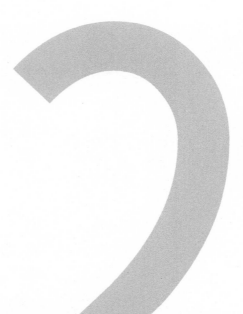

[86]

Questions! Questions! Old Grayhouse and a man's life? One man
I knew got himself a penile implant at 70. He had a purpose—
To keep it up, keep on doing it. It's always like that, every day,
To be a man. Am I long enough? Am I hard enough, thick enough?
Can I go down deep enough, last long enough, endure? Am I up for it?
Can I make her moan with pleasure, whimper with ecstasy?
Will I ever feel I've mastered the arts that please her?
Will she love me afterward? Am I worth something after all?

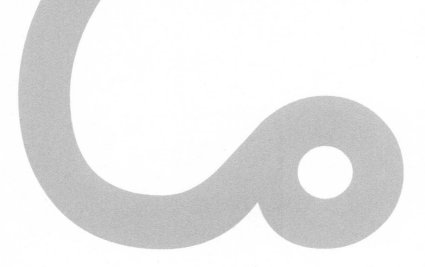

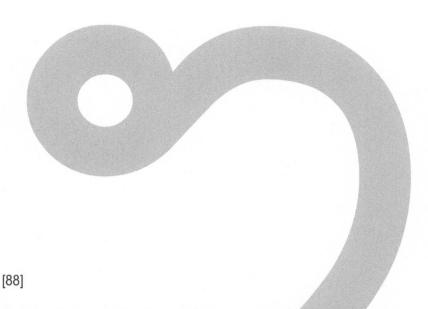

[88]

Well—at last—I'm dizzy, exhausted with these trumped up fantasies,
Grown bored with upturned regions for my cock or fingers to invade,
Of spreading thighs I wearily climb between, labia swollen or swelling,
Breasts both large and small, dangling beneath a woman on her knees,
Tipped with wine cork nipples or ripened olives. Sated with mirrored
Images of fantastic flesh, let me leave this last body lying on the sheets,
Fucked out, used up, worn down, killed with too much attention to detail.
Even my hair aches! Please, Muse, close your legs, let old Gray-house
    sleep.

Made in the USA
Las Vegas, NV
18 March 2022

45868437R00049